HAVE FUN
BE SAFE!

Paul Hotchopen

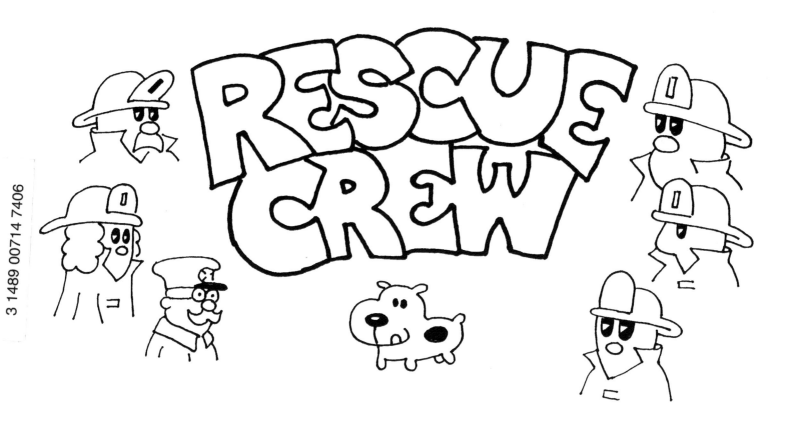

by Paul Hashagen
with Matthew, Sarah and Sean Smith, and Allison and Timothy Hassell

Published by Fire Books New York
20 Maryland Ave.
Freeport, NY 11520
www.paulhashagen.com

ISBN: 978-1-938394-32-4
Library of Congress Control Number: 2018943217

Printed in the United States of America.

First Printing

Produced by:
Great Life Press
Rye, NH 03870
www.greatlifepress.com

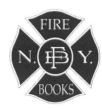

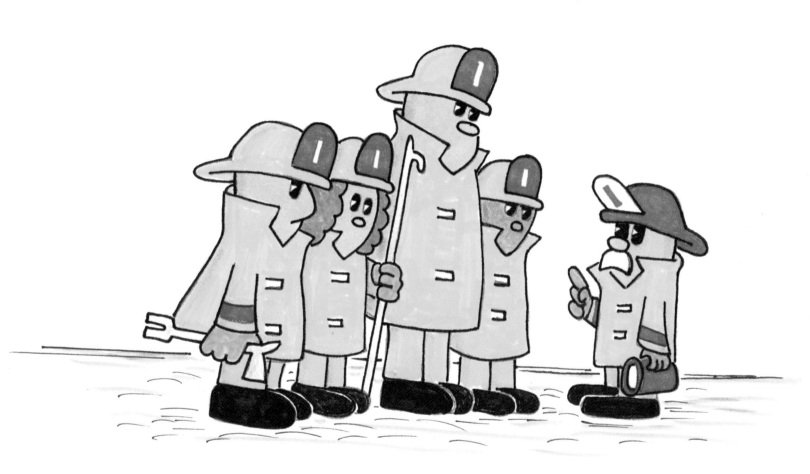

Our town has some brave men and women who work night and day
to keep us safe. They are called the Rescue Crew.

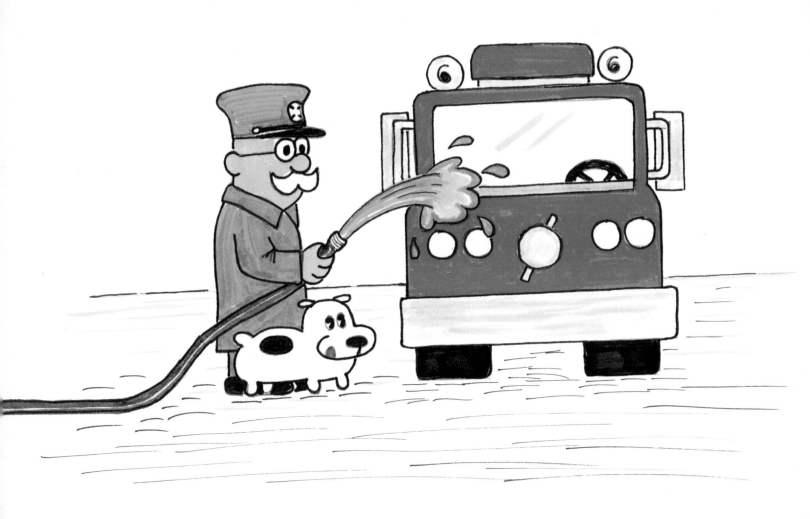

They have a rescue truck with hoses, ladders, and special tools.
The truck and all the gear is always clean and ready to respond.

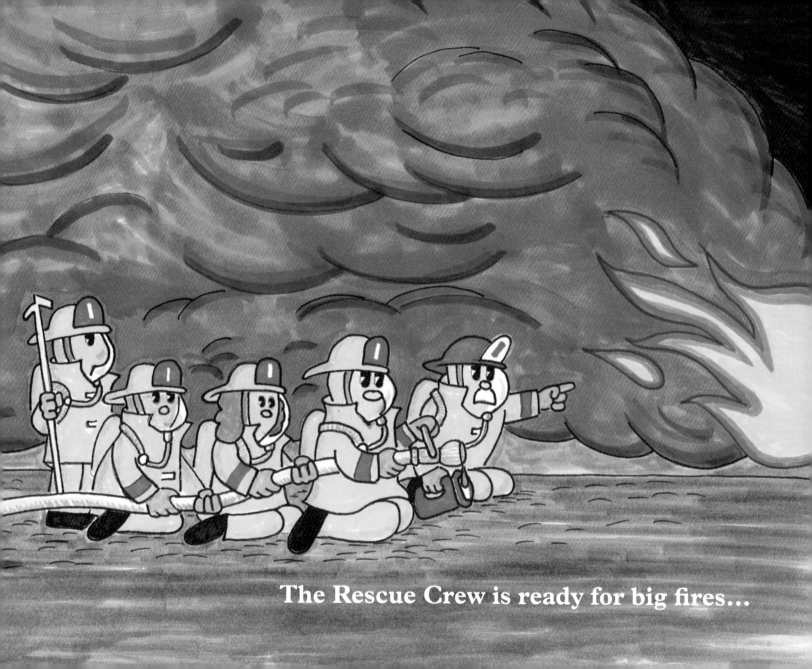

The Rescue Crew is ready for big fires...

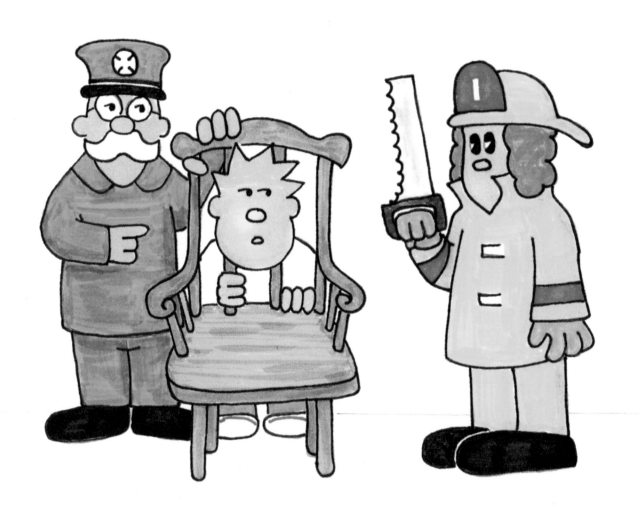

...or small emergencies.

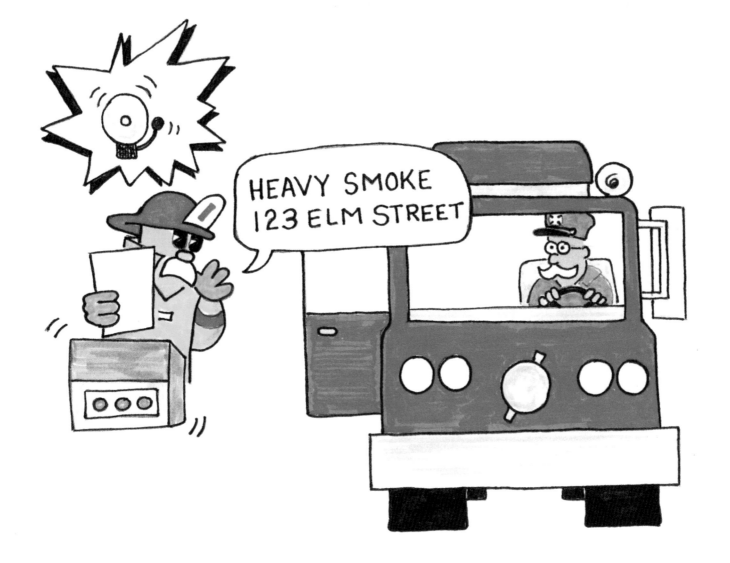

The Rescue Crew receives an alarm!

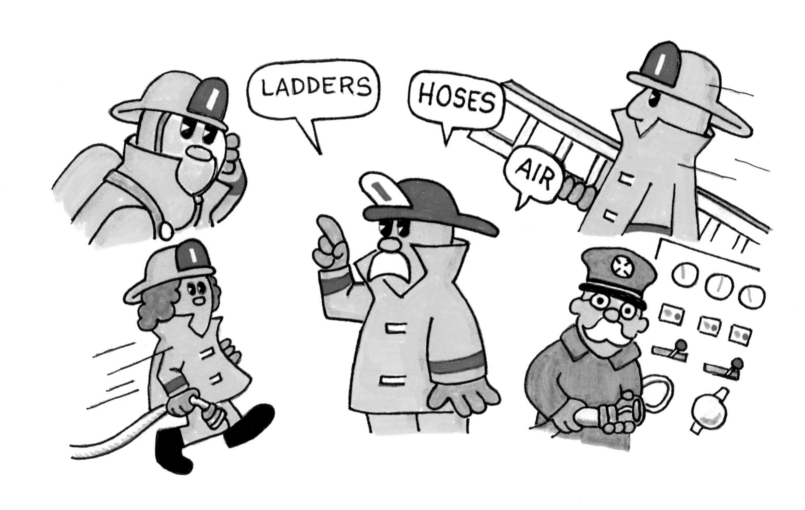

Captain Jack gives orders when the Rescue Crew arrives at the scene.

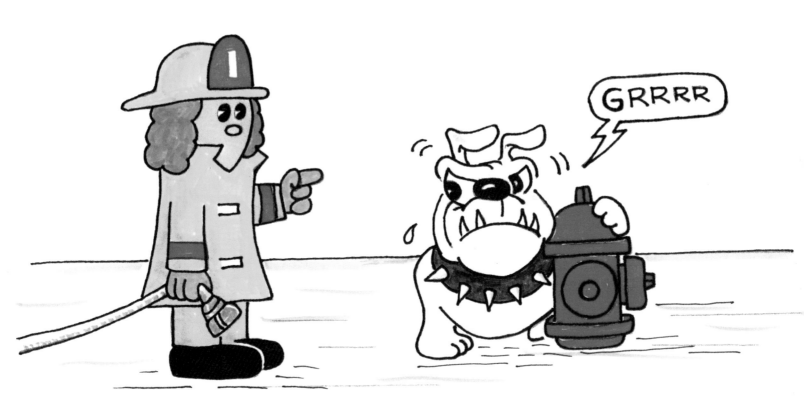

Ember has water problems!

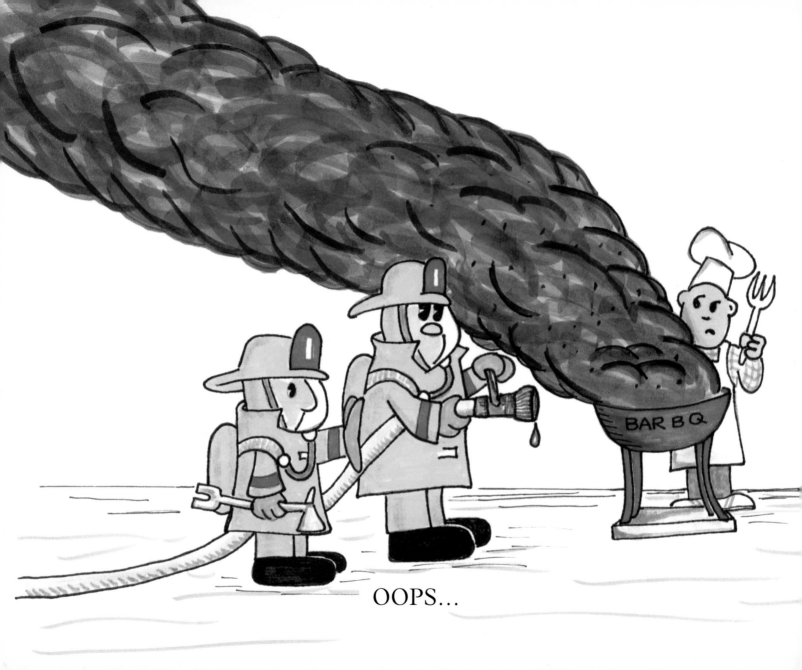

OOPS…

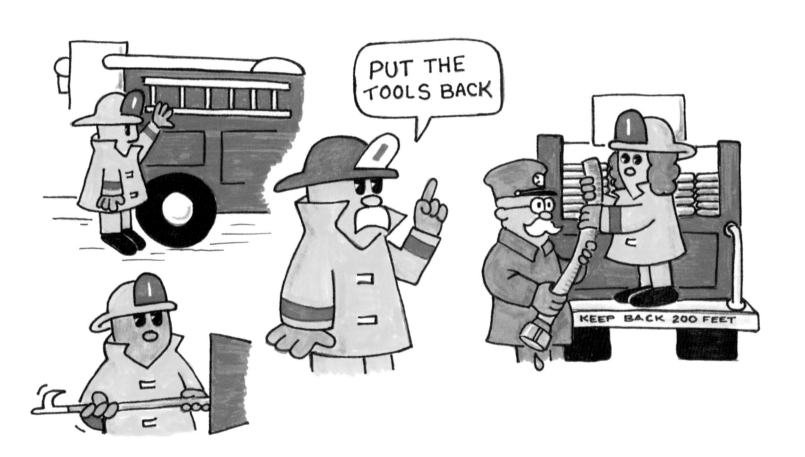

Captain Jack orders the Rescue Crew to get ready.

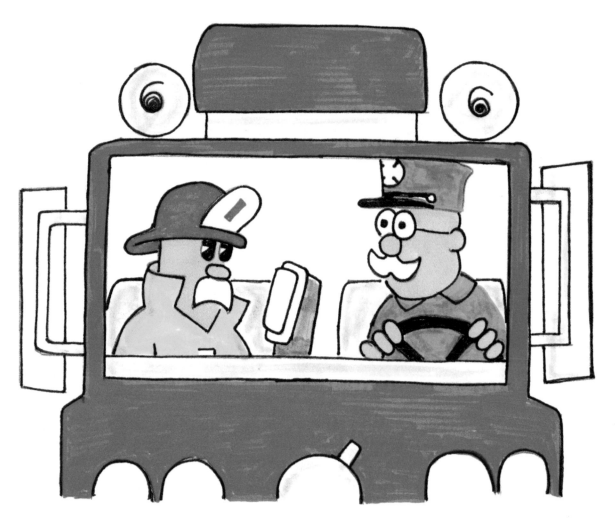

The Rescue Crew receives another alarm—

*Respond to the Oak Street School for a strong odor inside the building!

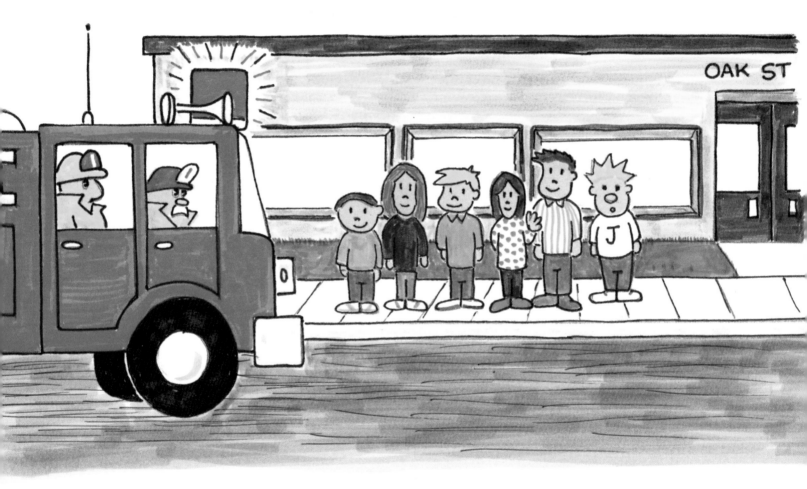

When the Rescue Crew arrived all the students were outside the school already.

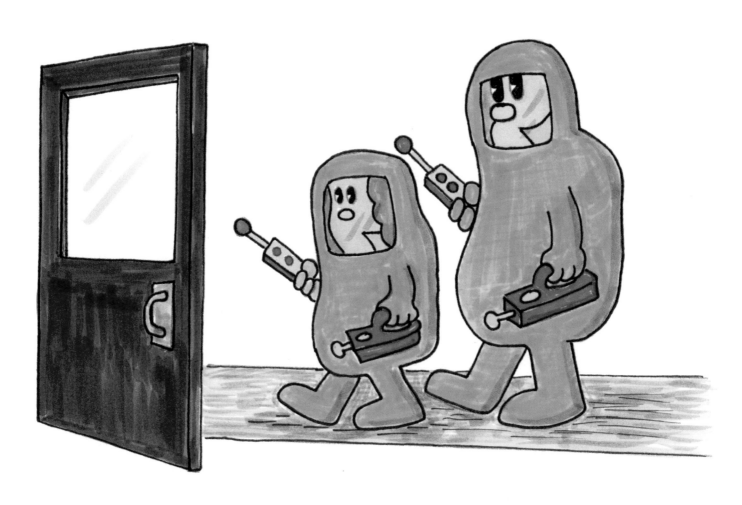

Ember and Shorty entered the school and searched for the smell.

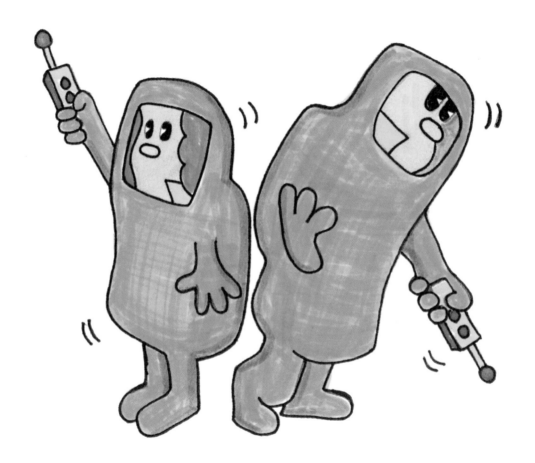

They searched high. They searched low.

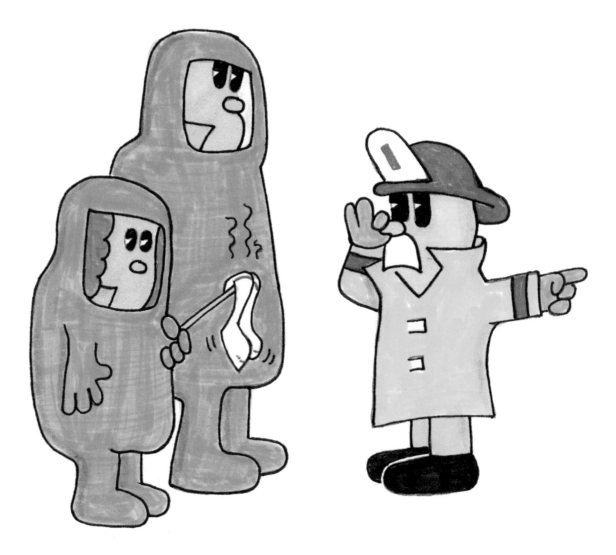

They found the icky smell. It was some old gym socks!

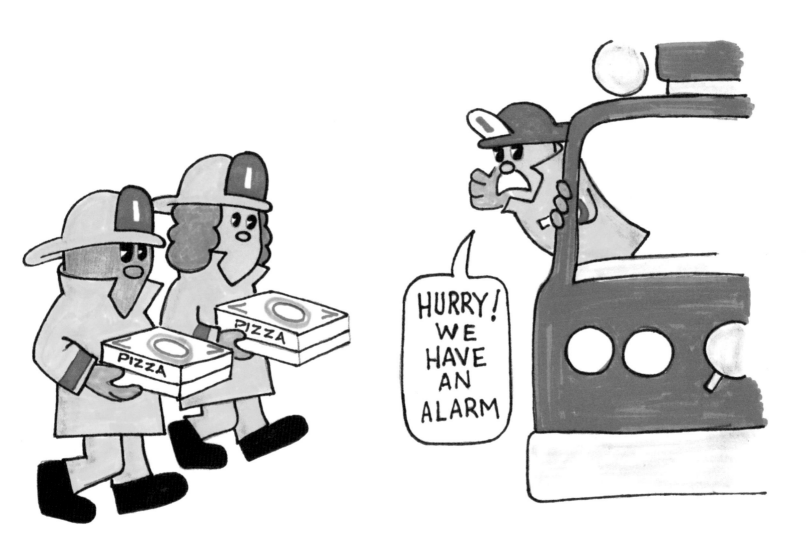

The Rescue Crew is always ready to help. Even at meal time.

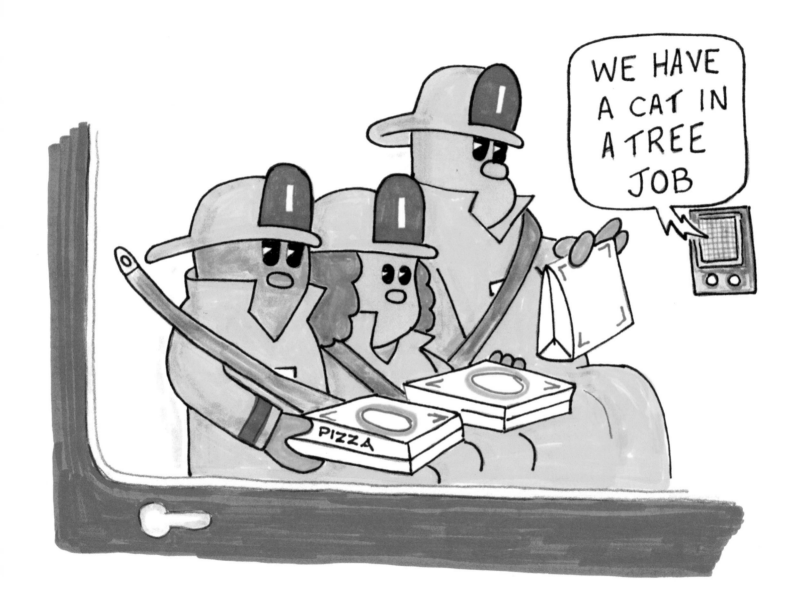

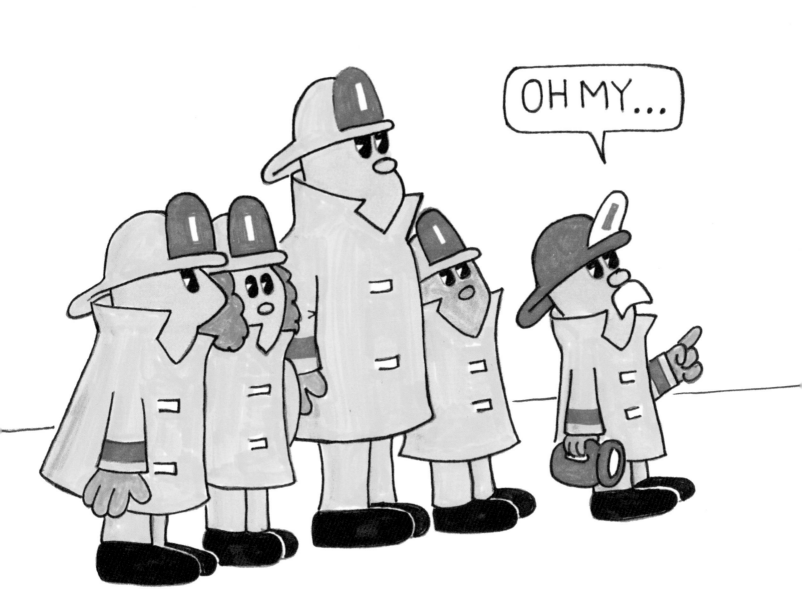

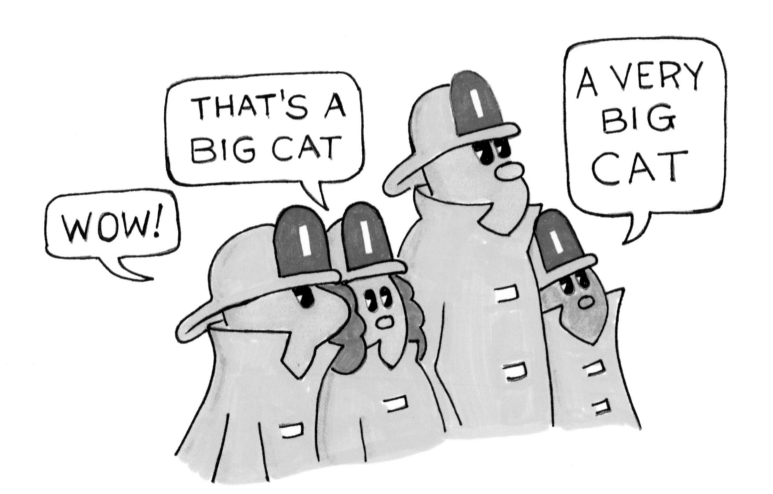

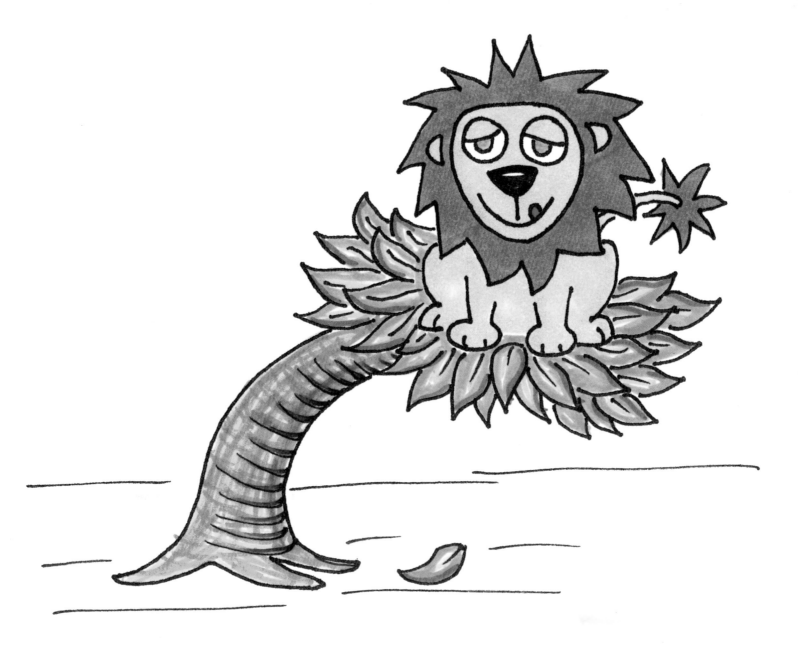

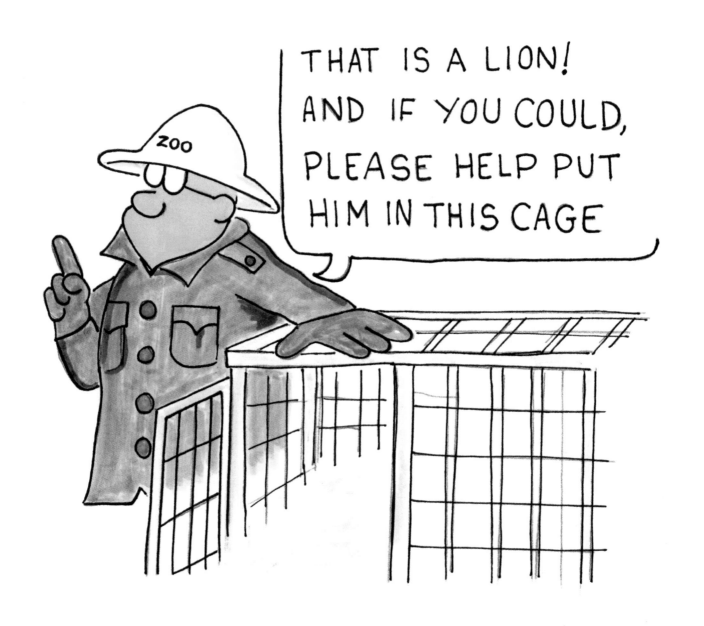

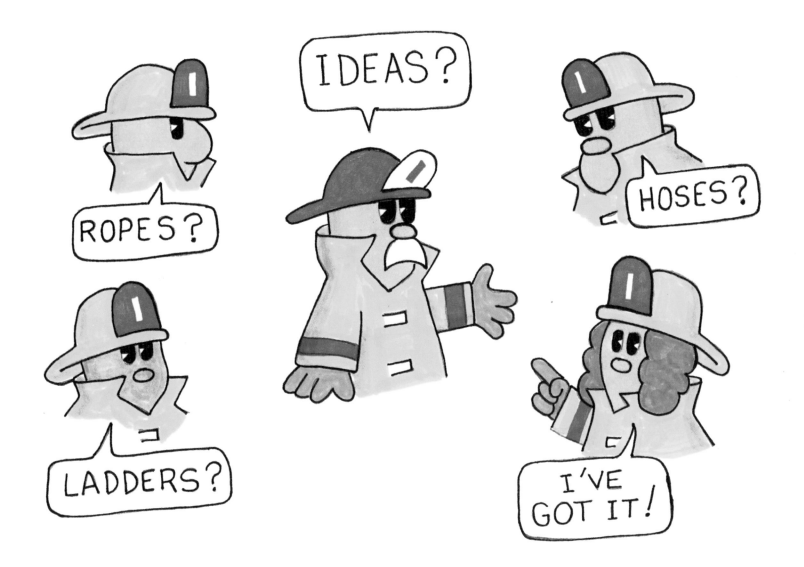

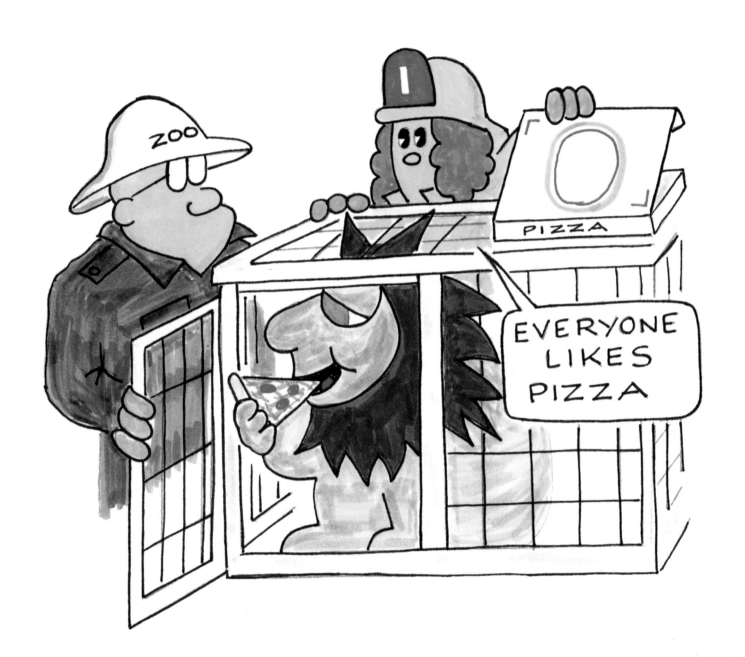

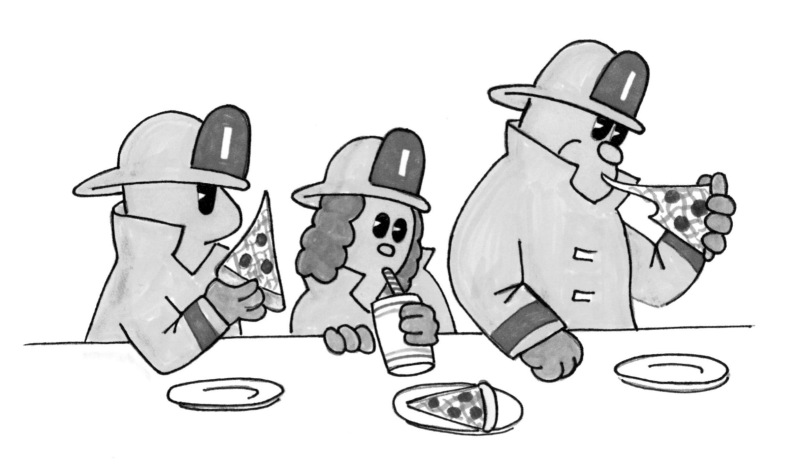

Lunchtime… finally!

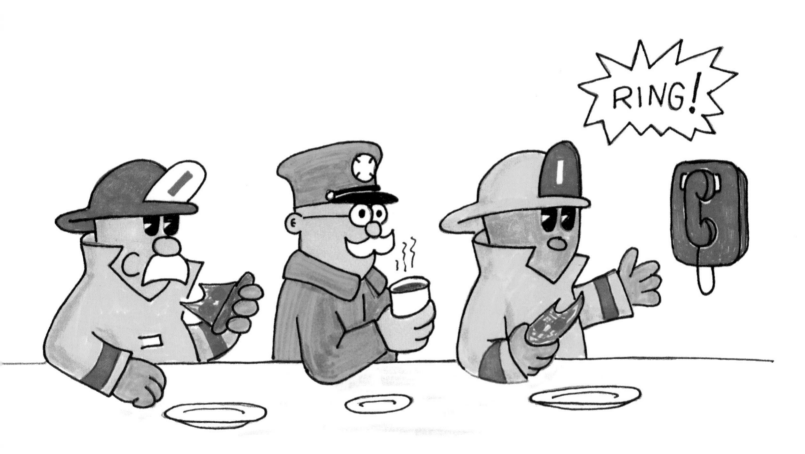

Then the emergency phone rang.

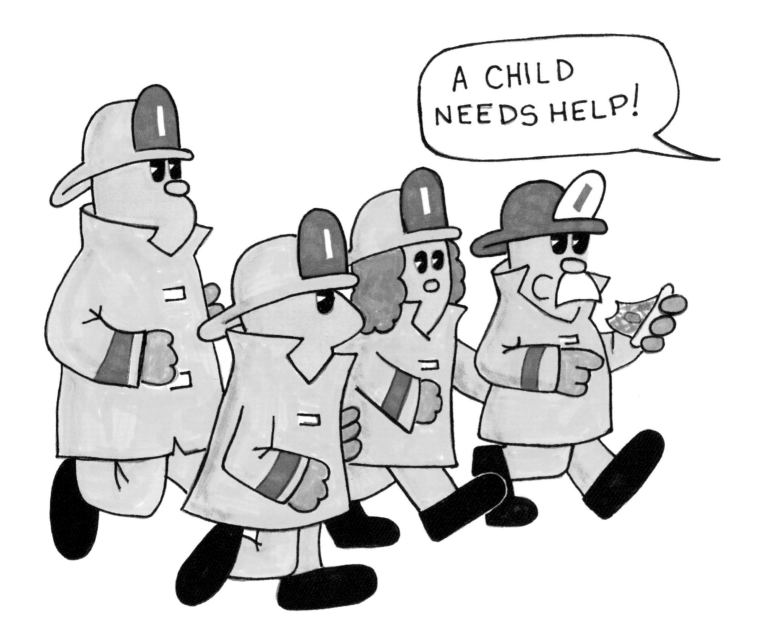

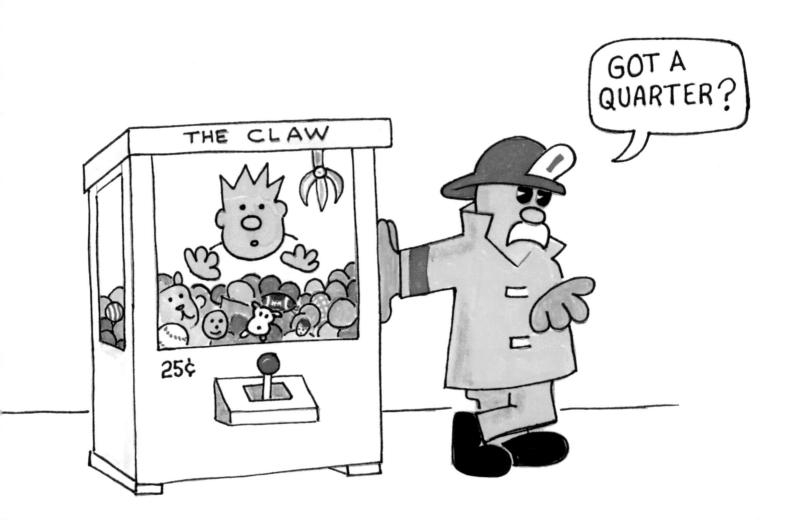

It was little Jimmy again. He was always getting stuck.

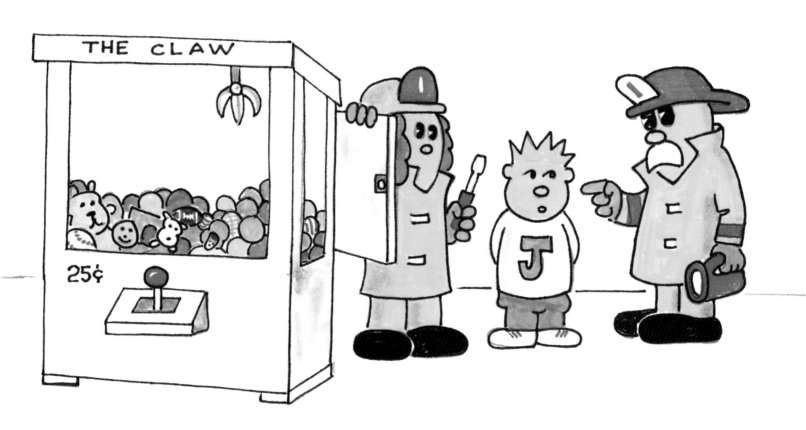

$2.75 later, Ember used a tool to open the back of the game.

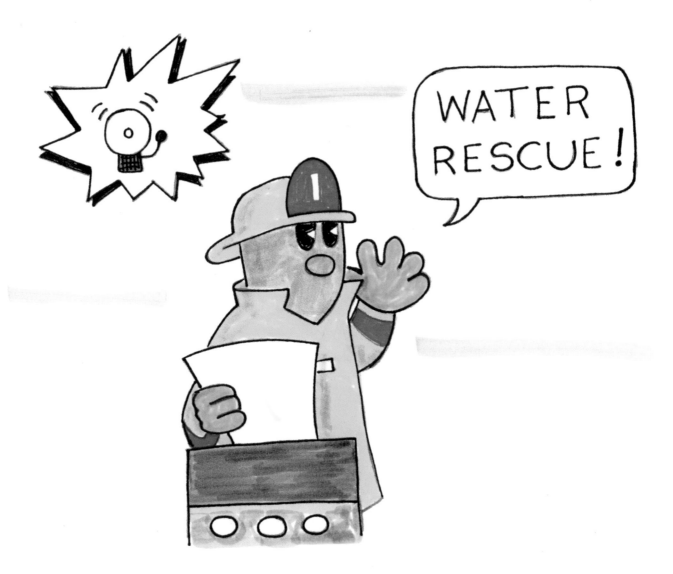

A little while later the Rescue Crew received another alarm.

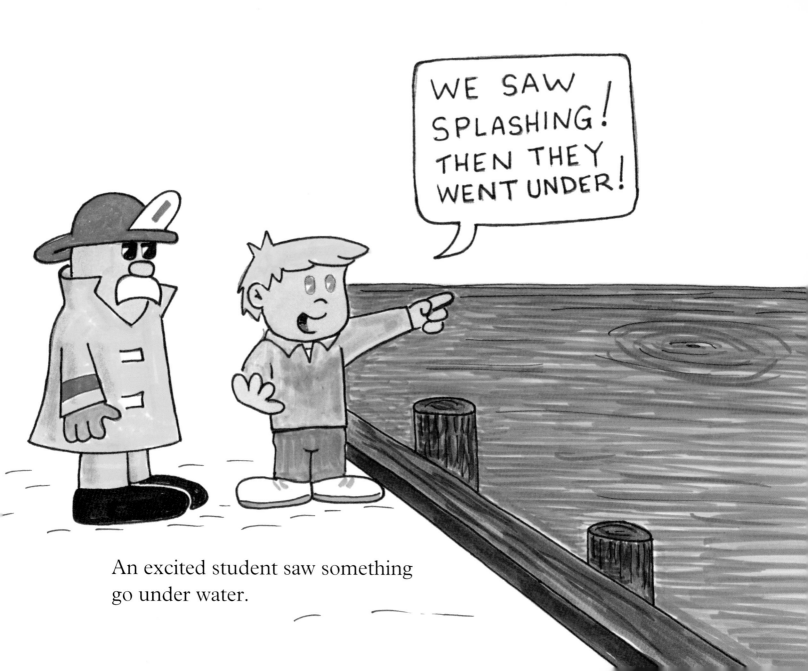

An excited student saw something
go under water.

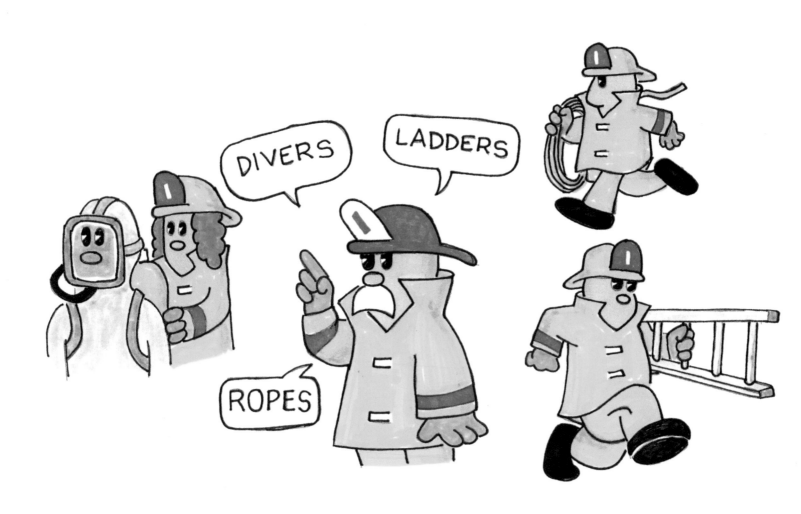

Captain Jack ordered an underwater search and rescue.

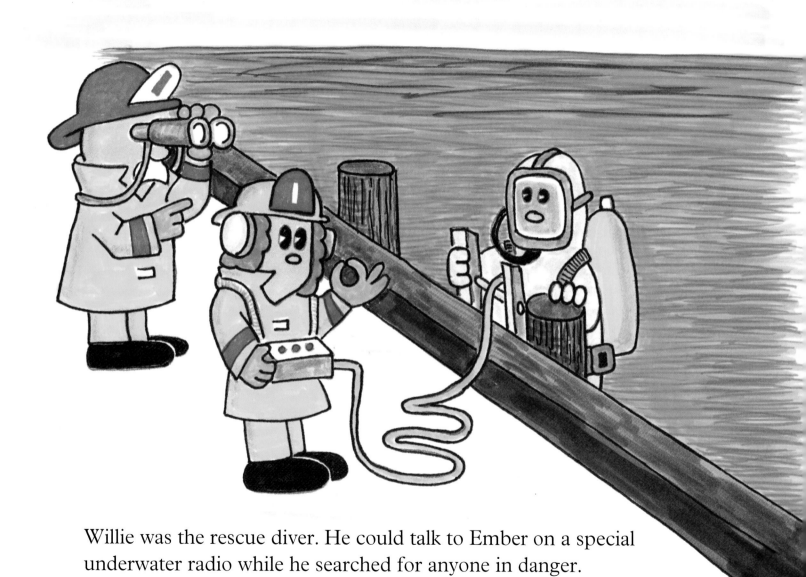

Willie was the rescue diver. He could talk to Ember on a special underwater radio while he searched for anyone in danger.

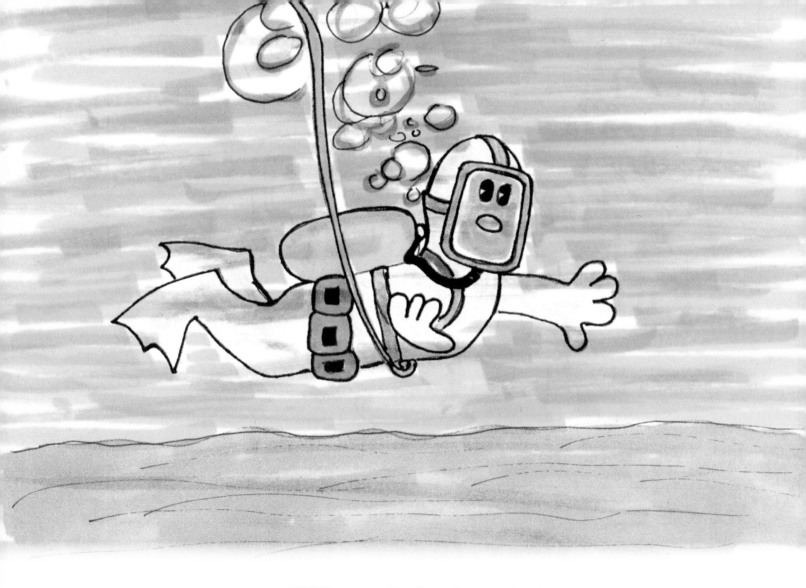

Willie searched and searched.

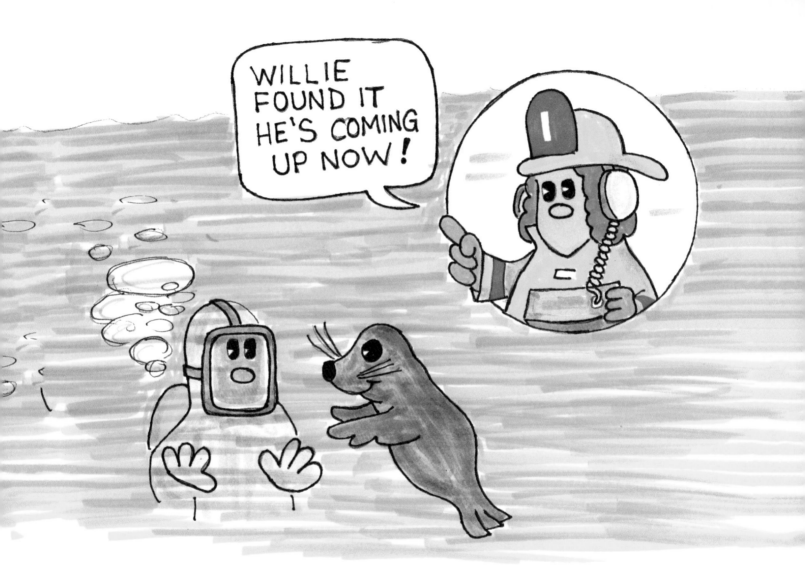

Willie told Ember he found something.

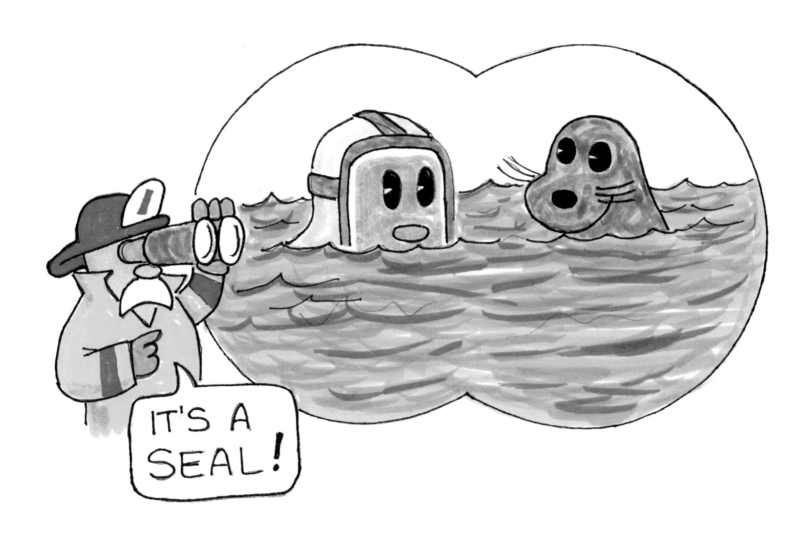

Captain Jack watched as they surfaced.

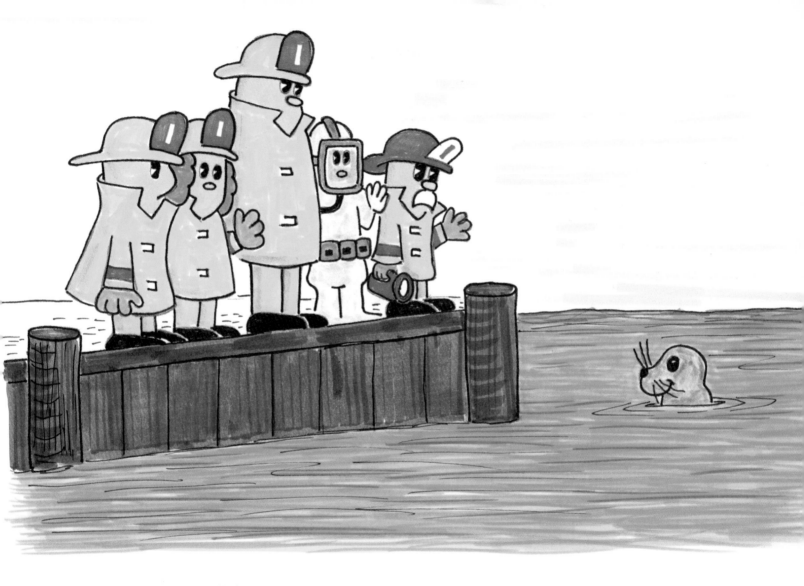

The seal was okay. He was just playing.

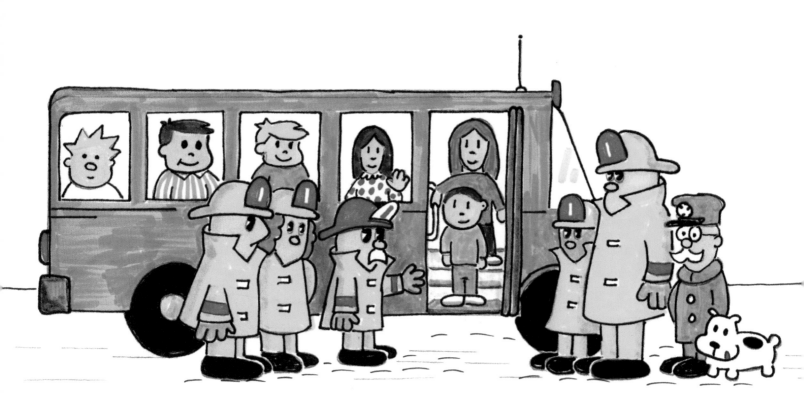

Today students visit the firehouse to learn about fire safety.

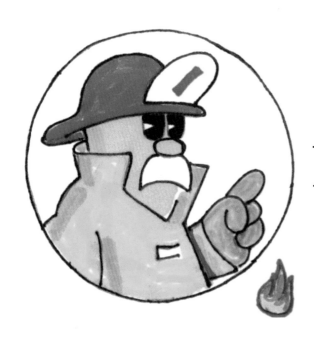

Captain Jack's Fire Safety Tips

Change smoke detector batteries twice a year.

Sleep with your bedroom door closed!
(Afraid of the dark? Get a nightlight!)

Plan Exit Drills In The Home! Practice escaping fire.
If there is an emergency Call 9-1-1

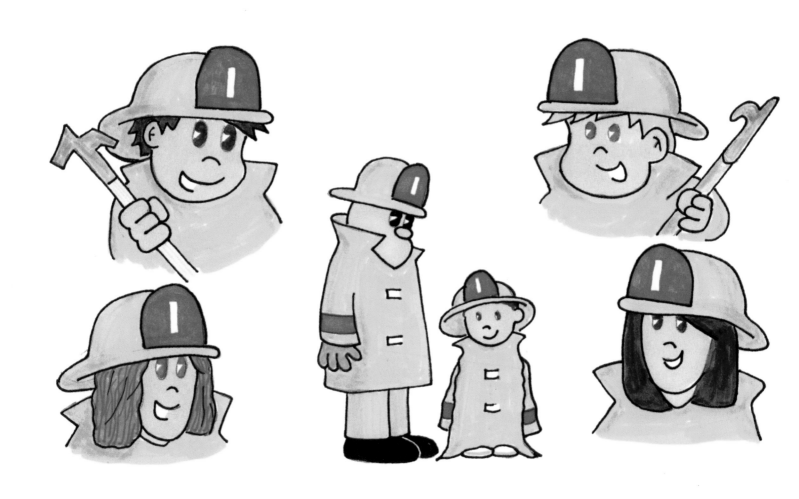

The students tried on fire gear and learned about fire tools.

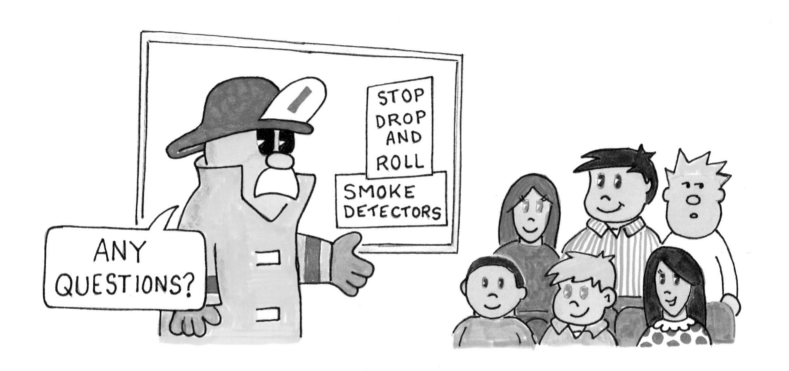

Fire Safety Day is <u>Every Day</u>!

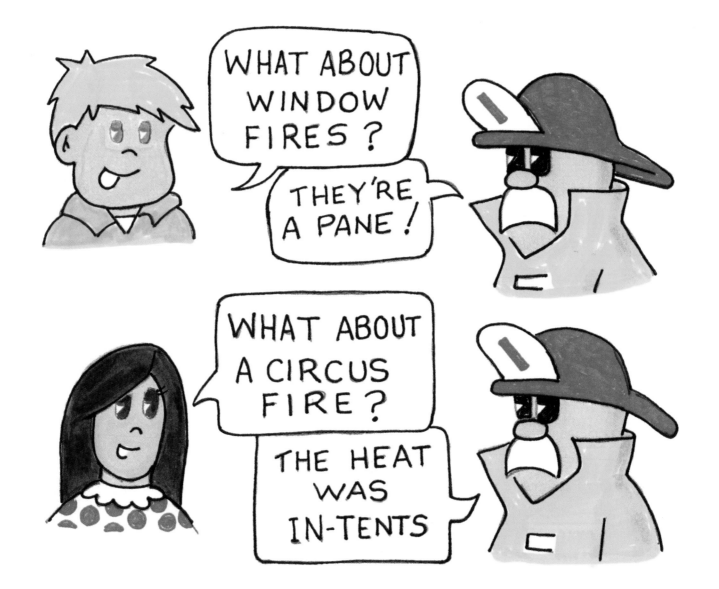

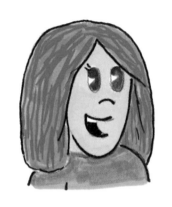
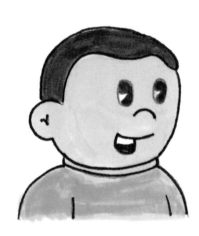
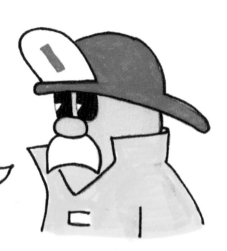
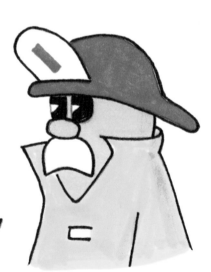

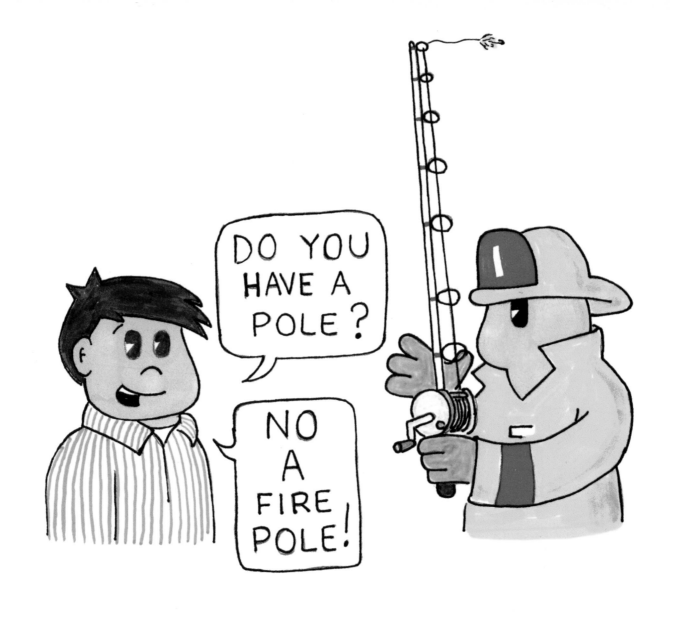

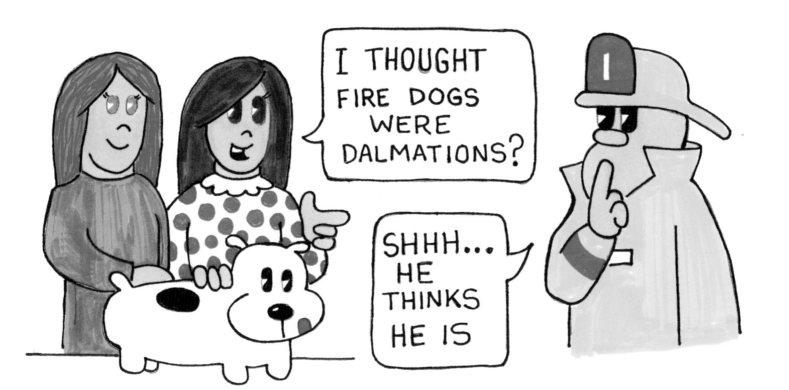

Dear Rescue Crew,

Thank you for letting us visit the fire house. We learned a lot. Thank you.

From,
Matthew

P.S
I think Spot is a cute dog and I can't wait to see him again!

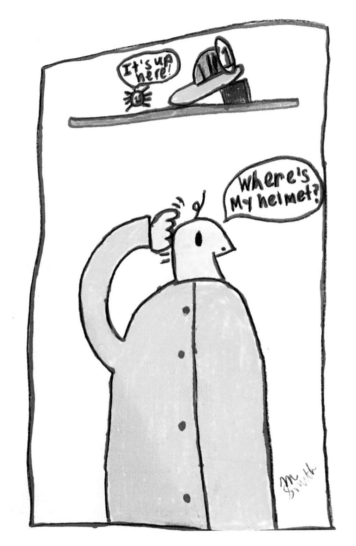

Dear Rescue Crew,
Thank you for teaching
us about fires and what to do
if there's a fire thank you.

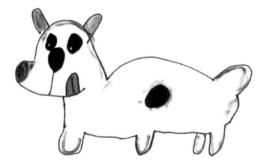

love,
Sarah

Dear Rescue Crew,
Thank you for teaching us about fire
fighting. I liked learning about how you
can use the rescue crews tools.

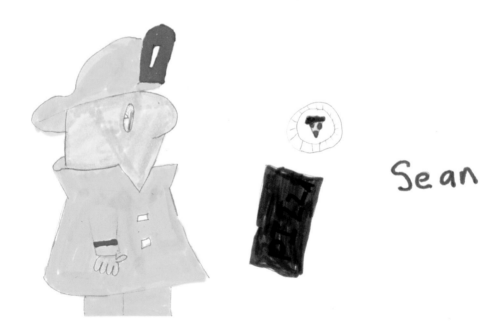

Sean

Dear Rescue Crew,

You are great! Thank you for being brave. I love how you saved Little Jimmy from the claw. Maybe next time he will be stuck in outer space.

Love,
Allison

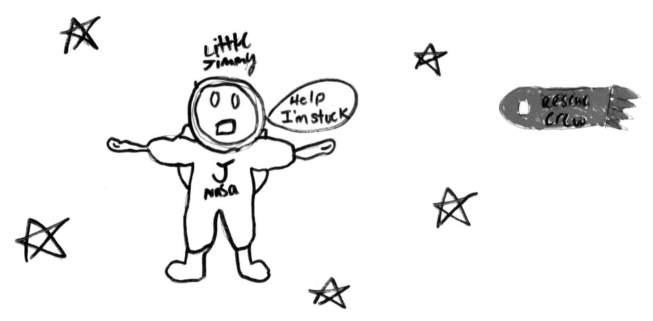

Thank you RESCUE CREW
for teaching me about
the tools you used
at the fire.

Love,
Tim

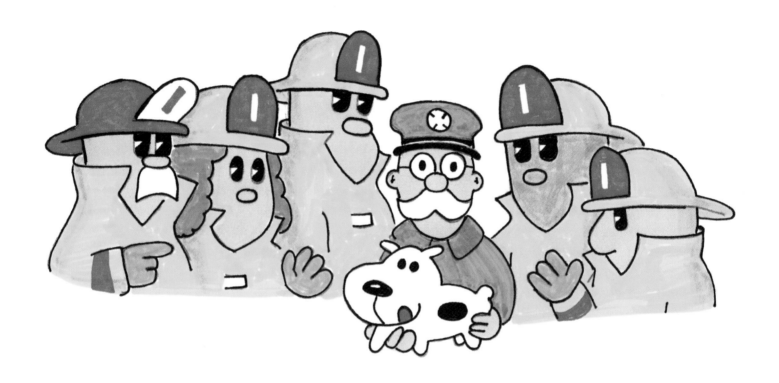

The Rescue Crew says, "Work hard, have fun, and be safe!"

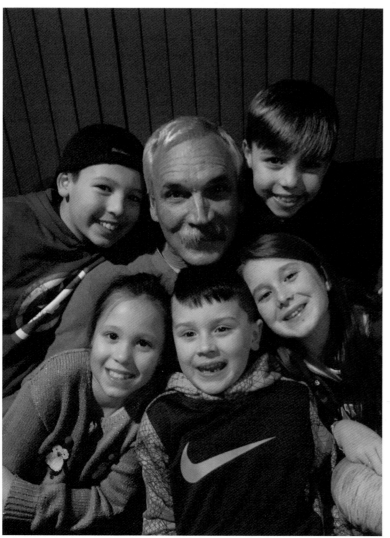

Paul Hashagen is a retired FDNY firefighter. His first fire cartoons were published in 1981. He has also written eight books on fire history.

Matthew Smith is a student and a junior black belt in karate, and likes to play video games.

Sarah Smith is a student and a junior black belt in karate, and likes to play softball.

Sean Smith is a student, and a junior black belt in karate and likes to play baseball.

Allison Hassell is a student and likes singing and dancing.

Timothy Hassell is a student and a fisherman, and likes to play football.

Rescue Crew is their first book together.